My Crazy Hotel Mates

CONTENTS

PART ONE

Where do I begin? (2000-2009)

PART TWO

INTRODUCTION

This is the second book in my trilogy, it is based on true events that I myself and my colleagues have encountered during our working life in the Hospitality Industry, the names of team mates have been changed and are completely fictious except for two very dear friends who are no longer with us. As a tribute to them they have been included as a special memory to all of us that knew them so we will never forget them. The story told paints a true picture of what life is really like working in the Hotel trade, it goes behind the scenes of daily life, the ups and downs from both a staff perspective and what the Guest expectations are. I hope it makes you stop and think when you next take a vacation that what you see has taken many hours of hard work to reach the standard that we all expect as a paying visitor. The proceeds from the sales of my book are being donated to Hospitality Action Charity to say thank you for supporting me through my illness, without them my recovery would have been much slower. The Charity do great work for all staff in the Hospitality sector ranging from Hotels; restaurant's, school dinners, bars and lots more they are a lifeline to so many people in difficult times.

Where do I begin?

It all started way back in the year 2000 when I desperately needed a full-time job after my previous employment was suddenly cut short due to no fault of my own. I went to one of those job fairs never expecting to find something that was about to change my life in the most unexpected ways imaginable, which would be the making of me. I was about to meet some of the craziest, wackiest, people from all walks of life, also the most loyal, lovable life- long friends from all nationalities. It was my destiny, my calling if you like! Never had I heard of the position called Room Attendant in my vocabulary, it was cleaner, what could it possibly entail? I was soon about to find out.

I arrived for my interview at a tall building that looked like a block of offices, no way did it resemble a Hotel especially from the out-side. Maybe it would be what I imagined when I got inside? Where was the posh bit like you see in the movies? You know the Ritz? All gold and chandeliers, Red carpet and such, no this was reality. With trepidation I entered what I suspected was the reception although it resembled a hostel and approached the lady behind the desk.

I explained who I was and was told to take a seat in an area to the side with little couch's or to me settee's, I was very nervous and wondered what on earth I could be letting myself in for when a small man appeared and introduced himself. We shook hands and he sat down beside me, surely, he wasn't going to interview me here? It was a bit public; I imagined being taken to a private room which was not the case. After what seemed like no time at all I was being asked when could I start? Wow! That was quick. The day after next was agreed, what on earth had I just done? I left feeling elated that I had just got myself a full-time job but also a little scared as I had never done this type of work before, oh well I didn't have to stay if it wasn't for me I would try it out, I didn't have anything else and I needed the money.
The day arrived and I entered what was to be my home from home for the next 8 years unbeknown to me.
I was a little nervous but more excited to have a look round this awesome building and to meet my new work mates.

After all the induction stuff to get out of the way I was itching for a tour me being a nosy kind of person, not much work was going to be done today, I should have savoured this moment because I wouldn't stop for the foreseeable future.

The Hotel had 111 bedrooms situated over 8 floors, lots of nooks and crannies, and two lifts for guests and staff which were placed side by side and stairs galore, seemed never ending to a newbie! Of course, we didn't go in every room just selected one's. The linen room, office, supplies of cleaning and guest products were all squeezed into one of the bedrooms that was no longer in use, very cramped, somewhere I was to spend many days and years to come. My head was spinning, so much to learn and to forget and so many new faces to remember, that was without the other departments and of course the guests. When eventually I was shown in a fashion what a room attendants job consisted of, in layman's terms the servicing of a room I did not think it was the job for me? First off the cleaning of a bathroom which was quite a decent size and the replenishing of the toiletries i.e. soap, shampoo, toilet roll etc. the folding of the towels which were to be placed on the heated wall rack and the washing of the floor tiles on your hands and knees! Ok you might say but each day you were expected to increase your workload until you reached the required amount and standards which was your quota for the day! Then add onto this the bedroom come living space.

The beds were a mixture of sizes, kings, Doubles and Twins, all extremely heavy to move, wooden bases, no casters that would have been too easy, back breaking if you did not bend correctly.

This was the housekeepers Achilles heel! The bedding consisted of sheets, Duvet covers and pillow slips plus the fancy little blanket which had to be folded a certain way, for use on colder nights. Now changing duvet covers is not everyone's cup of tea it is an art form in itself and requires lots of practice, the bug bear was getting them on correctly only to find a mark or tear which happened quite often, rejects has they were known in the industry, very frustrating having to repeat it all again. Then came the hospital corners which was also a required skill to make the beds look presentable and professional, I used to practise on my own bed at home the difference being your own bedding is soft, hotel bedding is starched to make it look good. Next was the polishing of all the dark wooden surfaces, after you had cleared out all the trash and boy did people make a mess, after all they presumed as they were paying why not? Dirty Devils! I often wondered if they lived like that in their own homes. Maybe if they had to clean up, they might think twice? Yes, they are the guests and are always correct! Last came the hoovering and the replenishing of the guest supplies so that they could have a well-earned cuppa! When you had mastered all this, you went on to the next room until you reached the grand total of 14 rooms. If your work mates had phoned in sick you got a bonus of a share of their allocated rooms what joy! Not many people stayed in this type of work for long it was more of a stop gap until something better came along, most chambermaids (old fashioned term) had bad backs and very sore hands due to the linen and chemicals. Then to add insult to injury along came the guests, now they were a breed all to themselves, nothing was ever good enough for them, you got the occasional lovely ones who were grateful for all your hard work, but the moaners and groaners came in all disguises. There were the posh ones who thought you was their personal slave and would have you fetching and carrying, the grumpy ones that would ignore you after you had said good morning to them when passing in the corridor you were not worth speaking to after all you are only the cleaner, and the perverted old men! Yes, there were plenty of those especially if young pretty girls were on shift. Last but not least those that believed paying for a room entitled them to all the stock off the trolley! (I'm paying so I can). I carried on in my role as room attendant for about a year getting to know my way around this vast place, learning the entire lingo, the sayings to get me in and out of guest rooms, breaking my back, yes literally! I was taken to hospital as I could not move even for a pee! The most excruciating pain ever all because I did not bend correctly when moving the damned bed; I had actually torn my groin and needed an injection. It was very common in this type of work, so I was placed on the sick first time ever in my employment. Staff came and went and eventually I progressed up the ladder to the position of Team leader, this now entitled me to not only self-check my own work but that of my fellow workers. I felt important with my new title and badge but I was now the one to blame if any complaints were made so I took my role seriously and put my all into it, now I could see what my colleagues were up to when cutting corners, some were disgusting even to my standards.

Let's just say always re-wash your cups and glasses before putting them to your mouth and please wash out your bath if you are unlucky enough to have one. The guests were just as bad, they came from all four corners of the world each with their own bad habits, those from the poorer countries had bad hygiene standards but they didn't know any better it certainly opened your eyes, the ones that wiped their bums and put the paper on the floor, sometimes in the bin, not down the loo? It wasn't their fault the sanitation was none existent back home, the smell was horrendous, it was normally the orchestras that were travelling around they occupied most of the rooms for a week or more, good for business when the hotel had a quieter period not for staff morale.

Getting in the rooms was a problem as they did not speak or understand English, when you eventually gained access the mess was unbelievable, you felt like crying. They would wander in and out of each other's rooms tuning their instruments, trying to communicate with you for supplies, getting frustrated when you didn't comply, we were lucky to have an assortment of staff that could sometimes help us out but only if they were on duty.

The bins in the bedrooms were the worst as they ate a lot of fish, Raw! The heads and eyes would stare at you and the smell? How we did not throw up I will never know? However, staff would go off on sick leave quite often around their visits.

The next groups would be the Chinese/Japanese they would visit on a regular basis, you were ok if you liked Chinese food as they were always cooking in their rooms even when told it wasn't allowed. They brought lots of cooking implements and what we could only assume was jars of strange pickles stood on all the surfaces, the housekeepers would all put their own take on what they were laughing and debating saying that the jars looked like they contained body parts. They were lovely friendly people with limited English, always asking me to come back for tea in their room with their families, of course this was not allowed so I had to decline gently, however they showered us with gifts of scarfs and plates beautifully decorated in fancy boxes, porcelain I believe, which I still have today. I need to get them valued! It still didn't make up for the mess that we had to clean up when they departed; the greasy smell would linger for weeks. They were very intelligent people and used the kettles in the rooms to boil eggs in, I had to make sure every kettle was inspected and clean before I could give the room back for sale, could you imagine another unsuspecting guest making a cuppa with a boiled egg in there? I wonder how many I missed.

The housekeeping staff did not have an easy job, many wet beds, who knows what from? You could only guess, plus they had a big workload in limited time as guests would be able to check in from 2pm in the afternoon, especially if existing residents were late checking out, or the ones that insisted that you clean their rooms now has they wanted to work, entertain or sleep.

That used to get my goat why would you want your bed making to get back in it? I'm sure it's not hard to throw the duvet back on, but no they have paid for service so want it now!

Then you got the ones that asked you to come in and service their room but would watch your every move (some were creepy) the girls were told never to work alone in a room with the door closed always wedge it open and if they felt unsafe get a colleague to work with you, some of the guests would only have a towel wrapped around them or little clothes on it made you feel uneasy. We as supervisors would be constantly checking to see if the staff were ok as only one team member operated on a floor and they were quite long and lonely. Then along came the swimmers and the professional ice-skating teams from all around the world, they were up and down like yoyo's and made the job extremely hard especially trying to fit around their very busy schedules. The swimmers would always want to rest and sleep in the busiest part of the day, as would the skaters who all rehearsed at different times, it was like a tip most of the time with lots of clothes, food and memorabilia scattered everywhere. The only good thing was the free show tickets that were allocated to the staff that made it all worthwhile, we also learnt a few good tips of how to pack a suitcase and live out of it like a well-stocked wardrobe, so it wasn't all bad.

The hardest part of the job was fetching your own clean linen and removing all the dirty, we were not lucky enough to have a linen porter, the staff had to drag the bags into the lifts onto the floor where they had been assigned, unpack it and load onto the housekeeping trolley saving the bags for the dirty when they had finished servicing a room, it was backbreaking work especially if you had extra rooms to clean and were located on different floors plus you were already tired at the end of your shift.

Some of the housekeepers would go up and down the stairs pinching off each other's trolleys has they couldn't be bothered to go all the way back down to the office especially if you were working on the top floor, this would cause squabbles between them as some of the staff were lazy.

The worst part was when the lifts were out of order dragging heavy linen bags upstairs was no easy challenge you were knackered before you started cleaning, throwing them down was better trying to avoid the customers this happened quite regular, I don't think the lifts were designed for such heavy traffic.

Talking of the lifts they were great when working but they did break down quite often especially when the hotel was full with large groups, the breakdowns would always seem to happen on a weekend when maintenance were not on shift, if you happened to be Duty Manager well that was a treat for you guests would often get stuck in the lifts between floors other than calling out the Fire Brigade the DM had to walk up the stairs to the top of the building climb out onto the roof, boy was it high and always windy, climb the rickety metal steps and get into the control panel to switch off the power.

I had a fear of heights and nearly pooed my pants when trying to climb back down, I couldn't do it facing forwards so backwards it had to be, then back down the public stairs to the floor where the lift had failed, to open the doors manually to release the terrified guests. If we didn't turn off the power and opened the doors, we could have decapitated the poor unfortunate trapped residents, I don't know about the customers needing a nice cup of tea to calm them down I personally needed a brandy.

I would rather have had a nice hunky Fireman rescuing me any day!

Next came an opportunity to climb the ladder as a vacancy had arisen for the Head housekeeper position, I was put forward as a candidate, but I was not all that keen it was a huge responsibility and I didn't know if I could handle it.

I am not a person to shy away from a challenge; my colleagues kept cajoling me to at least try as they didn't want a stranger to come on board, better the devil you know.

They knew my work ethics, firm but fair. I clinched the deal then my life took on a different meaning, lots to learn, new ideas, lots of training courses and mixing with the big boys, very daunting having to get to grips with all the red tape, living and breathing hotel jargon.

My home life had to take a back seat as I and others spent most of our time trying to make the hotel the best place since sliced bread, we were like one big family even with our little social time.

As we spent most of our time together lots of affairs between staff and management was going on behind the scenes, it was expected with having much in common and never going home, no one said a word it happens! Some did take it that one step further it is where you usually meet a partner after sharing most of your days and nights together, others fizzled out as people moved on or were forced to seek alternative employment it just would not have worked you shouldn't mix business with pleasure.

Staff were not the only ones, guests who were obviously playing away from home would book a room under an assumed name only for a day let, never appearing together, putting the do not disturb sign on the outside of the door, the noises coming from there gave them away.

The housekeepers would often find sexy underwear tangled up in the sheets which could not be saved in lost property! Used condoms under the beds or on the side tables why they couldn't dispose of them properly, disgusting!

Did they want to get caught? The nasty stains on the bedding which would sometimes leak through to the mattress which we then would have to scrub. The mattresses in most hotels leave a lot to be desired, usually very old and worn, bad stains from god only knows what, holes to make you shudder, but you as the guest were not supposed to look at this just the lovely bedding on top all pristine and white. You can imagine that they've had lots of bodies from all around the world doing whatever upon them? HUH! Better not go there!

I had to learn how to separate myself from my colleagues as I now was their manager and having to tell your friends when their work was not up to the required standard was very hard, but I had no choice as my own employment would have been put on the line. I worked alongside them demonstrating how and why things needed doing differently if we were to be the best housekeeping team around, it didn't always go down well and unfortunately some employees could not hack it so moved on to other employment.

I also had to let some go but I needed a strong and happy team. I was left pretty much to run the department as I liked if my targets were met, my standards were very high, and I earned myself the nickname of Hawk Eye! I suppose I should have felt chuffed as I could see what they couldn't. I did have a couple of supervisors whose job it was to fill in for me when I had meetings, training and precious time off. However, I always found faults, I suppose we all have our own goals to achieve, looking back the rooms were mine I knew every nook and cranny, each fault, so I took it too personal, but I was in my element as this was my dream job. I had always wanted my own little guest house by the sea so in a similar way this fulfilled my needs as the hotel also had a river running by.

The most challenging part of the job was being taught how to interview the general public in a professional way for housekeeping positions, it was very daunting even though I did have some training.

The language barrier was difficult as I tried to impart crucial information to a blank face not sure if they had understood anything I had said. After reading their c.v. (curriculum vitiate) looking for the most suitable candidate I then had to sit in a room asking questions awaiting answers when all I mostly got was yes, no, and head nodding with lovely smiles while all the time I was watching their body language trying to assess if they would fit in with the team.

Some were only attending because the job centre had forced them to keep their benefits. I grew quite accustomed to recognizing the shirkers that would waste my time if I thought they might be suitable I would offer a trial shift of one day where I would personally demonstrate the job in hand, cleanliness was the top of my agenda and I could usually tell after the cleaning of a few bathrooms if they would be the team member I was looking for.

 One such incident comes to mind when a young male told me a pack of lies about his work history he obviously had never done this type of work before after going back to check the bathroom he was just stood there not knowing what cleaning products to use,

I caught him cleaning the bath with the cups sponge it was such a mess he was nearly in tears and confessed that he didn't want the job and could he go home?

 I did offer to train him but we both knew it would have been fruitless.

At the end of a trial shift we would go to my office and sum up the day, I would ask them what they thought of the job and if it was what they were looking for, some would decline as they found it much too hard, others who were too slap dash I let go, better sooner rather than later, hotel work is not designed for everyone you need to be a grafter as its very repetitive and tiring and I would not expect anyone to do something that I could not.

Eventually I built up a great team where the turnover of staff reduced which made it easier to move forward with new ideas and more productive ways of working.

The team was made up of all nationalities, ages and genders that all brought different things and challengers to the group. We had fiery tempers who didn't like following new ways which clashed with others, some who were very territorial over what they presumed was their floor and didn't want to work anywhere else, the ones who took pride in their rooms and housekeeping trolleys who had a tantrum when another colleague had worked to cover their days off and had left it in a tip and not refilled the stock, which I did understand was most frustrating. The staff that cut corners then denied it who were forever getting sent back to correct mistakes, others who told blatant lies about not changing the bedding and covering their tracks by putting clean starched linen in the dirty laundry bags. This was instant dismissal if caught, harsh you might think but imagine the repercussions for the hotel if a guest caught something from soiled strangers bedding? The staff knew the rules but there's always one that breaks them and no amount of crying and sorry's got them their job back.

Catchy advertising

Back to the guests it was a day to remember and something I will not forget in a hurry it was mothering Sunday, a special day it most certainly was. One of my senior housekeepers came running to find me, "there's a strange nasty smell coming out of room 915" she told me "I cannot work it's making me heave" she said.

The first thought that sprung to mind was a death in the room; we all know that this could happen as the public used hotel rooms to commit suicide or something more sinister. "ok I replied I'm coming to investigate" my heart in my mouth, sure enough as I stepped out of the lift the smell was real bad getting stronger as I approached the room, but it was the smell of faeces (shit).

I knocked on the door shouting "housekeeping" no answer, so I used my pass key and slowly opened the door making my way in with the housekeeper behind me gagging.

The room was empty just the bedding all in a huge heap on top of the bed, my first thought was have the guests sneaked a dog in here? I tentatively started moving the bedding slowly, expecting to find a huge turd sitting amongst it, no nothing there, strange! Where's the offending smell coming from then?

The senior housekeeper had by now left the scene, it must be under the bed I thought to myself so I dropped to my knees and peered underneath, no all clear, well it's got to be in the bathroom but that would have been too easy, as I entered I noticed that the shower curtain was pulled across, oh no its something in the bath.

My heart was pounding as I slowly drew back the curtain not knowing what I was about to find only to see nothing, well it's in here somewhere I said to myself, by now a group of housekeepers had gathered in the doorway all eager to see what was going off.

Then a light switched on in my head the only place I had not looked in was the big wooden wardrobe surely not?

As I opened the door sat staring at me was the biggest dump I have ever seen it was more like an animal would do, donkey sprang to mind, was this a joke? Who would do such a thing? Did the guests not like the room? Was it a protest of some kind? All the girls wanted to look while I hot footed it down to reception to see who had occupied the room and to report the offence. As luck would have it, we still had a copy of their payment details so they would be getting charged for the cleaning and lost revenue of the room, but I mostly wanted to know why? The management did get in contact with the offenders it turned out that it was a couple and the male had problems (he certainly did) but are you telling me that the woman could not smell? They could have removed it, maybe she was immune to it. Well they wouldn't be getting back in the hotel in a hurry, that's got to be the worst Mother's Day gift I've received.

One of the main highlights for the room attendants was the lost property share out which happened roughly every three months so we could bring the stock up to date, all the spoils were placed in the office for everyone on shift to have a rummage for anything that took their eye, it was like a huge jumble sale it was fun but got a little tense if someone picked an item that another staff member wanted, arguments would break out and lots of bartering took place, all the unwanted stock was bagged up for the charity shop, you could walk away with some pretty decent stuff as it was amazing the things the guests left behind and didn't bother to claim back or they probably didn't miss until many months later.

 My team thought that I worked too hard and I needed a man (probably to sweeten me up) so the little darlings went behind my back and plotted to make me one out of all the lost property, (how they hid it I do not know) when I entered the housekeeping office sat on the laundry bags across from my desk was the man for me! I laughed until I nearly wet myself, it was genius though. We also reused him and turned him into a woman with a large bump when one of the room attendants was taking maternity leave. I liked to get the best out of my staff, it was a very heavy job and I appreciated their efforts, so I used to organize incentives with prizes to say thank you. We had an employee of the month award for the person who had performed the best, good timekeeping, went that extra mile, helped their colleagues without being told and most importantly kept good standards, they would win a meal for two in our restaurant on a night of their choice and be treated like a guest, it was well worth winning, the management thought it was a great idea.

The man for me and transformed into a woman

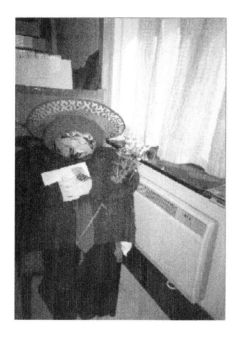

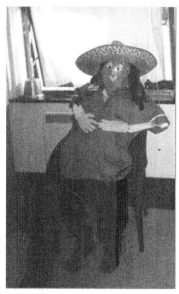
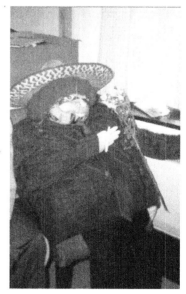

When Christmas time came the staff was encouraged to decorate their housekeeping trolleys keeping in mind that the guests would see so to make it tasteful and not tacky after all it was a hotel and not a grotto. One of my ladies used her initiative and strung fairy lights all around her trolley and used the plug on the corridor to light them up, cheeky!

The guests loved it. When the hotel started slowing down as we closed for Christmas day, we let the housekeepers finish shift early and treated them in the restaurant to a Christmas dinner with all the trimmings served by the management to say thank you for all their hard work it was lovely to all get together, we did a secret Santa where I would dress up and use a laundry bag as a sack and deliver the gifts it was a perfect wind down, not many hotels closed on the big day but we were an independent company so didn't have to follow others.

We also had annual awards where all the hotels, restaurants and supporting venues competed for the best of the best and the unsung heroes of hospitality. It was a great night out where management and staff who were chosen mixed for the evening all dressed up to the nine's for wining, dining and entertainment it was the event of the year and we all wanted our places of employment to win, it was nerve racking also as they played your entry interview when you was placed under pressure so you gave some silly answers, it was great fun for the onlookers who were supporting you, you gave a huge sigh of relief when it was over, we were all very competitive and wanted to get an award.

If you were lucky enough to win you had to go up on stage shake hands and have your photo taken while your teammates all cheered loudly.

After all the presentations the evening would continue with dancing and drinking into the small hours many sore heads the next day if you were unlucky enough to be placed on shift.

Back to the lovely guests, we had lots of sickly one's that had either over-indulged while dining because their companies had paid an allowance so why not take advantage? The one's that had been on an organized evening out where there was a free bar so you could imagine the consequences later that night when they arrived back to the hotel (must have been the air & taxi ride) some did not make it back to their rooms the hotel reception was a number one spot, all over the fabric chairs and carpets as if a knocked over bottle of red wine wasn't enough. When they did manage to get upstairs the night staff had a nightmare with drunk, out of control guests trying to get into other visitor's rooms causing chaos, urinating on corridors and the lifts. This is hotel life where the police were called many times during the night for unruly residents.

Then along came the ladies of the night that were either called to the hotel or smuggled in, if only the walls could talk? Also there was the crazies to contend with at least two types, you got the ones that would shout, run up and down the corridors banging all the doors disturbing others they were often evicted or fell asleep in some strange places, the morning cleaners would stumble over them.

The other crazies well what can you say? For example, someone had a fixation with post it notes and literally plastered them all over their room WHY? Then left them for the night porter to remove, what were these people on? Next were the domestics, you would often think someone was being murdered with all the screaming of obscenities and crashing and banging why people brought their troubles for all to hear, probably liked the attention.

The night porters had a job and half and saw many sights. The days were just as bad, one that springs to mind was when my young male room attendant entered a room of a guest who was staying on, and these were called remakes.

A very well to do business lady (not so sure lady was the correct term) had puked up all over the bed and floor she had the cheek to go about her daily routine without reporting that she had made a mess and was sorry, no poor Tom was expected to clean up after her.

What would she have done on returning to find it still there? It beggar's belief. We must also not forget the guests who believed that they were too posh to flush! Why would you leave it for the chambermaid?

It's bad enough having to clean the toilet, people had disgusting habits.

It got worse if the customer had toilet problems with loose stools and would pebble dash the entire area, or ladies on their monthly's and leave blood smeared all over the seat as if the bedding wasn't enough, yes we know it cannot be helped and loo brushes are not provided due to health and safety but you would at least try to clean up or contact reception for some cleaning items, they are aware that the room attendants are both sexes, but no they are the guests and expect waiting on hand and foot.

On occasions we were short staffed, so it was all hands-on deck that included reception and sales staff, well that was a shock to some of them, I found it highly amusing when a large group were on the way and the previous occupants had just vacated due to a late check out. Some of the reception staff had helped before it was the sales staff, and no I wouldn't have been able to do their job! We had one lady who was lovely, but it nearly killed her, it's a totally different world servicing rooms and under pressure you need stamina, after one room she was flagging and asked for a break to get a drink, "no way "I told her "we don't get tea breaks up here" her face was a picture she said I was a slave driver, I don't think she ever volunteered again.

Every residential building had issues that did not seem to have a cure for problems that occurred out of our control, this one was not exempt, it was situated close to a river, not a very clean one at that, not somewhere for swimming in if you get my meaning, and after all we are the steel city.

The hotel had a problem with spiders inside and out some big beauty's at that plus their cobwebs, as fast as we tried to get rid of them more would appear we were forever chasing them especially in the public toilets down the back staircase, we got used to them in the end we had no choice it was shut your eyes and try not to look, makes your skin crawl.

The hotel was built like a tower block which I don't think it was ever intended to be as it had a petrol station built underneath how did it ever pass the planning and safety laws it was beyond comprehension it was a tragedy waiting to happen, before the smoking ban came into force we had two smoking floors plus customers and staff would stand outside front and back having a quick fag break it just never entered our heads how dangerous it was? One near miss that's been brought up often was the day a reception staff member had a waste bin on fire she ran with it to the petrol station to put it out WHAT! WHY? That could have been the end of us all.

Another date that was to become a day that unbeknown to me would have a significant meaning for the rest of my life was the 11th of September 2001. I was checking the rooms after the staff had serviced them when I came across one of my ladies on the 9th floor just stood frozen looking at the television screen it was the start of her shift.

The staff were allowed to put the tv on for background noise and also to check if they were working correctly, she beckoned me in to come and have a look, it was the unfolding of the terrorist attack on the twin towers she was visibly shaking, petrified and believed we could be a target. "please can we go home, I don't feel safe, I don't want to be here, what if a plane is coming to smash into us?" she said "we are too high up I'm going downstairs, are you coming with me I don't like this." I was just about to try and console her when the second tower was hit, this was frightening and I too wanted to run, at the time it was not clear what was happening in the world. Could this be the start of a massive attack on all the tall buildings? Nowhere appeared to be safe, not even travelling home, how we got through the day I do not know, it must have been the quickest shift we ever did. I would not have liked to be a guest staying in such accommodation that day it must have been very frightening. The date was to reappear 13 years later when I underwent emergency surgery for a life-threatening brain tumour, I was one of the lucky ones as I survived 9/11 the poor people trapped in the twin towers and planes did not stand a chance.

Life moved on, the hotel went through many changes, new owners came on board with different companies providing new products, laundry changes, staff relocation it was exciting as we were now part of a chain, we had more to learn, new training procedures plus more money to spend on new items that we had been crying out for.

 New mattresses at last it was like a military operation getting the old ones out as they fell to bits, very heavy to move, floor by floor, my team was set up to remake all the beds, exhausting! We even had new mattress protectors it was like Christmas.

Then came new curtains, carpets etc. but one thing that didn't change was the guests they were still challenging, they didn't like the new beds too hard, un comfy, made them sweat, just needed something to complain about, yes and they still soiled them. We still had the hen parties and stag do's boy what a mess they would make it was alcohol fuelled so we didn't expect anything less.

One weekend I was duty manager we had a group of lovely men that turned into animals after drink, they had to leave a bond before we allowed them to stay, when it was time for checkout I was called to inspect their rooms for damage before releasing it.

I knew that Sunday morning when they staggered back into the hotel much the worse for wear with little or no clothes that trouble was ahead, they disappeared to their rooms, I was hoping that they would sleep it off, no such luck, the party continued with myself having to tell them to quieten down as other residents were not impressed, I could not get into the room they all seemed to have gathered in I found out why later.

When coming to check out I did the room inspection and boy had they made a mess, broken kettle, coat hangers, beds upturned, broken bed slats, beer bottles, cans, lots of rubbish strewn everywhere, takeout boxes with pizza, kebabs and such rubbed into the carpet and what looked like chocolate sauce smeared all over the mirror and TV screen utter chaos, why did they think it was acceptable to leave a room in this state and to get their bond back?

We would not have been able to clear the mess out in 20 minutes never-mind service it for re-sale. When I told them they could not have their money back they started pleading with me that they needed it for transport home, no way was that going to happen, eventually we made a bargain I would get them some cleaning supplies and they could jolly well clean up all the mess and I would check it to make sure it was done properly, they went back up-stairs with their tails between their legs to be quite honest they did an ok job, I kept a small amount of the money for breakages but they got to go home, that was a stag weekend to remember!

The night porters had the worst ones as I said before, the night manager was on reception while the porter kept doing his rounds to check that all was well up on the floors, especially when all the drunken guests arrived back.

One evening Joe was doing his walk about when he could smell faeces (shit) very strongly on one of the corridors, he searched behind the fire-doors, lobby etc. but could not find it, he knew it was there, the only place he hadn't looked was the lamp-shades on the walls to light up the corridors, you guessed it stuck in one light shade was a turd nicely warming up with the heat from the bulb, you wouldn't believe it, he took it downstairs to his colleague who was not surprised it became known as shit-shade. On another occasion he had to turf out some unruly guests after many complaints from other residents to the noise factor when he got inside the room he could not believe the amount of sex toys all over the place they had been having an orgy he boxed them all up for the manager.

Nothing shocked them anymore even finding dead people either through natural causes or police investigations or suicides you had to have a strong disposition to do the job.

My ladies and gentlemen used to think the rooms were haunted when they learned of a death, they did not want to work on that floor said it was ghostly and that bins moved on their own and had a nasty cold feeling it was all over- imagination of course. Then we had the celebrity's and soap stars that stayed with us and because they were used to being waited upon, their rooms were very untidy, we did not drool over them just treated them like a regular guest, not making a fuss, I don't know if it was what they expected in fact I remember shouting at one famous lady for stepping on my wet lift floor after I had just mopped it, I bet that made her feel special? My staff consisted of all different ages, we had a good working relationship but unfortunately people moved on, left to have a baby, or to start a different career, the hotel started getting into difficulties, rumours started going around that we were going to close down, we went into administration and things were slowly going downhill, staff that had been working there for a few years were looking at other employment and moving on which put us all on edge. I too made the decision to apply elsewhere I did not want to be unemployed, I loved my job it was my second home and it tore at my heart strings to have to give it up but I could not miss my chances when they came along.

The day came when after 8 years of highs and lows I said goodbye to the remaining staff, part of me wanted the new adventure but the other half was sad to be leaving all that I knew and loved, all the hard work and dedication that had been put into the place, we promised to keep in touch although we knew that wouldn't be very often as our new life would take up most of our time.
I remember with great sadness on returning to visit my old colleagues at a later date bumping into one of my old housekeeping team members, she was coming out of the lift, a beautiful smile on her face as she recognized me, we exchanged a few pleasantries, had a hug and said the usual take cares, she told me how much she missed me, it was to become unknown to both of us as the last time we would ever meet as a few weeks later she was murdered. Such a lovely sweet lady taken much too soon in such a tragic way, one person who made such a lasting impression on my soul, never to be forgotten, her name was Weronika beautiful in every way.

MOVING ON

The next Hotel I moved on to was a 4 star 95 bedroom establishment, it was the year 2009. Now this one was what I expected it to be, it had a red carpet and chandeliers in the large event room. I was nervous, excited and a little unsure a bit out of my depth if truth be told but it was a new challenge which I was going to embrace. My Title was Housekeeping Manager which meant this time going in at the top; I knew it was not going to be easy especially with an existing team already in place who were probably going to give me a tough time. I needed to be firm and assertive but also not to just jump in feet first as I needed to get a feel for the place and assess my new surroundings.

The bonus being I had the management behind me, my role was to pull up the standards and take the hotel forward, some of the staff would fight against me as I was a stranger on their turf so I did expect this, it was not going to be easy.

After all the induction criteria, the show round, meeting the heads of other departments, getting my uniform, keys etc.

I was then able to have a closer look at my office where I would be based, the vast laundry room and boy was it big compared to the previous hotel, stock supplies which were greater due to the rating of the hotel, last but not least the guest rooms and the lady who was holding the fort until I was put in place. I had previously had a quick tour of the building when I was being interviewed I noted then that my work would be cut out if I was lucky enough to get the position, now I have got the time to look more closely it looks like a bigger challenge than I first thought. Not one to be deterred long hours and elbow grease were the first steps to getting the place how I liked it. Next came the job of sorting out my team, re-training staff one to one, this did not go down well as the ones that had been there long haul liked the way they did things and did not like change and myself so made it blatantly obvious, not to be beaten I called staff meetings explaining what was going to happen whether they liked it or not so they could either work with me or start looking for alternative employment as I was going nowhere, I had been brought on board to bring the hotel back up to standard and I had no intention of quitting.

Eventually I built up a great team, we all worked hard together. The rooms were very large compared to the last hotel with lots more items including mini fridges, gowns and slippers, lots more toiletries, bottles of water, different teas, more to forget until I got used to it.

The bathrooms were tiny hardly room to swing a cat very compact, the only thing that appeared to be the same was you guessed it the guests, still with dirty habits, demands, moans and groans.

This hotel operated room service, which was new to me, lots of food trays on the corridors, in the rooms all with half-finished food and drinks on them plus lots of empty alcohol bottles, i.e. beer and wine and ice buckets with glasses of all shapes and sizes some knocked over with spillages on the carpet what a mess and smell. On the upside it was a no smoking hotel but that did not deter some people who would put socks or plastic bags on the smoke detectors installed in every room, little realising when setting off the alarms the fireboard behind reception could pin point which room had triggered it, some very disgruntled residents especially if they were woken in the night and had to vacate to the car park in the pouring rain! It also had air-conditioning, which was a novelty, fantastic when it worked but a nuisance if the guest could not operate it or were too impatient to wait so would open the windows which obviously made it work harder so was less effective.

My job was very hard and tiring and I desperately needed a good supervisor who had knowledge of the hotel industry as I had many more tasks to attend to including Duty Manager shifts which were mostly weekends once I was trained up, this included covering reception lunches, it was very daunting and I made lots of mistakes.

 One I can remember which will haunt me was the car park barriers that needed a code to operate well me being a newbie at this could not work out were the bleeping was coming from

 I thought the computer was on the blink or the pager was being activated I just could not find out where the noise was coming from until the human resource manager walked past and I voiced my concern, apparently it was the screen at the side of reception with a phone that on the other end was an irate lorry driver stuck at the barrier pressing and pressing the inter-com waiting to get out and I was completely oblivious "shall I pick up the phone" I said, the HR lady replied" you had better not just open the barrier, he's not too happy" it's a good job she was passing, any longer and it could have been interesting OH WELL! We all have to learn.

The Job of housekeeping Manager had a lot more to it than people thought; I was responsible for all the 95 bedrooms, public areas, laundry control, Guest supplies, cleaning and hospitality stock plus lots more.

 It was a very demanding position you had to love this type of work if you wanted to stay on top, the hours were long and exhausting, you were on your feet most of the day, before the rooms were given back to reception for resale they had to be checked for cleanliness to the highest standard, this was a feat in itself especially if some of your staff cut corners, it involved running my hand around every bath if it showed a white powder then the girls had not washed off the chemicals just sprayed and wiped, the best ones was the big dirty rim all around the bath which I could see as soon as I looked behind the shower curtain, telling the housekeeper to come back and clean it properly was time consuming they knew I wouldn't pass it so why did they keep on pulling a fast one?

The excuses made me laugh, lost their sponge, run out of cleaning supplies, cannot see it, when I checked their sponge it was bone dry it hadn't seen water in a long time, did they think I was daft? It did not save them any more time so they should have just done it in the first place.

I had to peer down every loo the amount of times that they had left toilet paper down there then told me that it had been cleaned; what with I wanted to know? Some of the dirty habits they pulled when they thought I wasn't looking was unbelievable, one lady actually spit on her hand to wipe off a sticky mark on the bedside cabinet after I had told her to go back and clean it properly, it was acting like a naughty school girl being defiant no concern for the guest at all, I've seen it all.

The bathroom floors was where most of the staff tried to evade cleaning as it meant that they had to bend and get down on hands and knees, they missed the corners and round the toilet bowl always lots of pubic hairs stuck to the tiled flooring, I caught those that for some reason could not crouch down using a hand towel and shoving it round with their foot, it was the same when hoovering they only did the middle, corners did not exist?

The bedrooms too had their own problems, mugs on the hospitality tray always with stains inside, not enough replenished stock, missing milk portions, bedding with marks and tears hidden obviously thinking I would not check, dust on surfaces that you could plainly see and dirty torn information leaflets not replaced. I know that the housekeepers are on a time limit but if the room is especially trashed then we do account for that, time can be saved on a stay over or a please leave my room. My supervisors would often start off good but as you get tired, they would get slacker in their duties often just peering in the room not really checking it was a very mind boggling, boring, repetitive position.

Doing this day in, day out drove you mad it was nice to have a distraction like a blocked toilet when the hotel was full and no maintenance on shift bodge job here we come, out would come the wire coat hanger and a large plastic bag to cover your hand so you could have a good feel around the u bend not for the squeamish, the toilets were always breaking as guests would be too heavy handed or had been over indulging the evening before.

The laundry room was another vast area to contend with, all the linen, towels, table ware and there was lots, kitchen cloths, oven cloths you name it we needed it, the stock had to be unloaded out of big wire cages that would often get stuck we had to use anything heavy to bash them to get the lever open, the linen was heavy, packed in clear plastic, slippery, all needed counting and putting on the shelves in the correct places, the dirty linen put back in the cages and pushed outside under the awning.

The cages were heavy and did not wheel very easy, the worst part was counting the dirty festering oven cloths and sorting them out into the correct bags, they were minging, (stinky) warm, mouldy you have never smelt anything so bad all on an empty stomach, the table linen with lots of party decorations that fell out all over the floor and bits of food all stuck together, lovely; Then came the soiled linen which had to be bagged separately you name it we had it, this is what the public do not see, we don't just walk around with a little feather duster like in the movies, trying on guests clothes, this is the nitty gritty part of the job.

We had lots of different guests from all walks of life, Monday to Friday was the corporate business people who mainly stayed in the executive rooms, the coach tours that were touring the peak district mainly elderly and from other countries some with limited English we had to consult the coach driver if we had issues that couldn't be solved.

Weekends were mainly the families going to weddings, events, wedding parties themselves,

all congregating in the interconnecting family rooms situated on the 3rd floor running from room to room for makeup and hair and photography an hive of hustle and bustle, beautiful to look at but very frustrating for the housekeepers to go about their daily routine, plus very hard to service the rooms having no idea what to tidy up or remove.

Ideally we would leave until after the wedding party went out but some of the guests wanted to stay put while we tried to do the best working around them, probably to make sure we only touched what was appropriate for example wet dirty towels, used cups, glasses, etc. I only used to put my experienced staff on that could self-check to make it more efficient.

The next day when the party vacated, we needed a strong team as the clear up was very time consuming no one wanted to work on that floor willingly the staff certainly earned their money.

The beds in this hotel at least had castors but the biggest beds located in some of the rooms that I've ever seen called super-king, which basically consisted of two beds joined together by zip and link, wow I thought to myself how do you get the duvet on these without falling inside it?

Not many people liked them as they said they used to roll over in the night into the join, ideal for large families wanting to share a room plus when large sports groups were staying, we could split them. We also had roll outs now these were a pain in the bum most of them were past their best and would not wheel, very hard to manoeuvre from floor to floor and extremely bulky to store taking up a lot of space, mostly used at weekends.

The suites were best as they had bed settees in the living space plus a dining table and chairs, large flat screen television and a fridge, they resembled a little bed-sit. The best of the best, used mostly as the wedding suite, champagne on ice, fruits of the season, chocolates, balloons in fact fripperies to suit the occasion, we used to dread cleaning up the confetti and the rose petals that were scattered on the bed on valentines night, they went everywhere and usually took days to get rid of them.

One thing that never changed when opening the residents rooms first thing in the mornings was the stale pungent smell of feet and morning breath after being cooped up all night, you were lucky if you had an early riser who had showered and freshened the place up HEAVEN!

As most people are aware the first port of call in a Hotel is the Reception Desk, it is usually staffed by the younger generation eye candy after all who wants to be greeted by an older, mature person it's just not done, up and coming springs to mind, all the complaints are aimed at the receptionist so you need to be thick skinned and adept at solving problems in a professional manner while keeping your cool. It is a hard job as the general public can suddenly turn into monsters if things are not going their way, Arseholes is the correct term behind the scenes as everyone wants something for nothing or an upgrade! They are expected to have a world of knowledge of all that goes on in and around the hotel and beyond, we do not have a concierge as such so the porters double up to fulfil the guest's needs.

One of the biggest problems is breakfast, most residents believe that their breakfast is included in the room rate which is not always the case, it depends on who has made the booking, some web sites have an all in package and some need a separate booking, always bring your correspondence with you for proof or at least double check when you check in to avoid confusion the next day.

The worst ones are our customers from overseas with no English in their vocabulary its near impossible trying to make them understand, they will show you their booking on their mobile phones but it's in their own language so we are still none the wiser, doing hand demonstrations is quite comical but when you have a large gathering it's not an easy task, when you ask for their room number you may as well be asking for the next weeks lottery forecast as they just nod and smile and hurry along their way.

The General Manager was a little eccentric but a great guy he would roll up his sleeves and muck in when the going got tough, We used to have a 10.00 o'clock daily meeting with all the Heads of Departments Monday-Friday to discuss what events were taking place, what special guests would be arriving, making sure we all had enough staff on board to full- fill the days agenda, it was a great way to start the day.

We could also voice any problems that would occur as we were each given a turn to speak out, one of my queries was concerning having the pager when it was my turn to be Duty manager, the hotel had a spa and leisure pool, I could not swim so what use would I be in a drowning situation? Admitted the pool was shallow but it was still daunting on my part if I happened to be the only one around if called, it worried me greatly. Adam, who was a bright spark, said "Just throw all the floats and lifebuoy in and hope for the best" everyone laughed as they do!

I was just getting used to the GM when it was announced that he was moving on which happened in hotel life and a new company was coming on board which meant many changes some good, some bad, it normally resulted in lots of staff changes as a new broom sweeps clean, getting rid of all the dead wood! New Managers liked to choose their own staff after they had settled in, so we were all wary of what was to come.

New brands appearing, new items, new rules, lots of rumours going around, hotel life never stood still if it went stale you lost your ratings it was a very nerve-racking time wondering whose job was safe. The day arrived when our new General Manager was introduced to us, we observed him and likewise, he seemed ok, very quiet but like us all it was a new position for him, and he was weighing everything up. He didn't look the type to stand any nonsense, not forgetting he too had a boss above him, but it quickly became aware that he was not a people person, you were never going to become his friend.

In fact most of the staff were replaced one way or another even those who had many years' service it was a very upsetting time I wondered what on earth had I done changing jobs but it was too late now, he was just unapproachable, ignorant at times as though you were worthless, barked orders at you, not many staff got along with him only select ones that had been chosen by himself.

I was actually one of the lucky ones due to me having a brain tumour that at the time I did not know off, my memory had got affected which made me very confused as though I had got dementia, Oh how I would have loved to have been a fly on the wall to see all the things I was doing, it saved my job as no one could get through to me, I must have been a thorn in the managers side as everything just went over my head.

The guests still believed that paying for a room entitled them to take away as much as they could carry when departing, maybe they liked souvenirs of their stay, they would take the complimentary toiletries, biscuits, tea and coffee sachets, milk pots, bottles of water, notepad and pen, slippers (which were thrown away if used) and Dressing gowns, now these could be bought if needed but stealing them was better must have been the logo?

Staff too would inch these when leaving their employment, sewing kits, shoeshine mitts, in fact anything not nailed down would be considered some even took the little cushions with the brand name written across them.

Of course, we knew who was last to occupy the room so when challenged they just denied any knowledge of seeing the items, people like freebies!

It was the same old same old with the staff just a different building, we had lots of different problems to try and solve trying to please everyone which was impossible, not many people liked working weekends but it was a must in this industry as it was our busiest time, I tried to share out the days off as fair as possible but there is always one that doesn't play ball and upsets their team-mates, arguments would break out I would have to step in to keep the peace, nothing worse than bitchy women.

Then we had the staff that would not change their ways and would cause trouble thinking they had the upper hand until I took them aside and had a quiet word, they would sulk and act like children doing the job slap-dash making it harder for themselves. Personality's clashed, some were removed after a period of time, it was very challenging. We had good times too we often went for tea at the local pub to get away from work and let our hair down, team bonding. At Christmas time we all went for a meal and drinks, I would buy each one a little present to resemble their personality we had such a laugh, we played games such as charades and took up one corner of the pub it went down well, we were well known to the establishment.

Most weekends I was the Duty Manager in the mornings until the Restaurant Manager came on shift at 3pm and would take over to do her stint, it was always us two we would laugh as I always got the car break in's and she got the drink fuelled revellers, both of us had large departments to cover besides taking on this extra responsibility, I think I was on first name terms with the local police officers and the car repair services, I had my own hot line.

It was a joke, it was the invention of the sat nav where people stuck them in their vehicle windows, it was like a magnet to the local youths they were like magpie's, only smashing windows to get access which obviously made it difficult for the owner to travel onwards, it was a damn nuisance we ended up putting signage on display in the car park warning guests to remove them before coming into the hotel. There was also the fire walk to do which was a tour all around the building checking all the fire points with a machine, also the fire doors making sure they were properly closed.

I used to incorporate room checking on my rounds trying to kill two birds with one stone. I also used to miss my lunch in the staff canteen as show rounds had been booked to show perspective clients all the events- space we had to offer for their special birthday parties, weddings, christenings etc. It was a lot to take on, if a medical problem arose you usually were called to deal with it as we were first aid trained, it should have been a separate job not part of your busy department.

The night manager along with the porters saw many incidents amongst the guests often resulting in the police being called, mostly domestics that got out of control especially if alcohol had been consumed some people just could not handle drink.

The more serious ones involved those who not only fought between their- selves but also caused so much noise with the crashing and banging while smashing up the room that other residents were also afraid for their safety and would phone reception to ask for assistance, they would congregate out- side their rooms trying to find out what on earth was occurring, sleep was out of the question.

No one wanted to get involved it just was not worth it better left for the professionals, put it this way none of the offenders were going to be spending the rest of the night there.

Then came the sleep-walkers or so they claimed, one night the evening manager was doing a bit of catch up with his correspondence at the front desk when a mature small female appeared in only a little top and knickers she beckoned him over to say she had just woke up from her sleep walking and could not get back into her room, obviously she hadn't picked up her key card when she went on her little jaunt. "Do you know what your room number is madam" he asked her "yes" she said thank goodness for that thought the night manager,
 he had visions of walking around the hotel with her scantily dressed trying to find out where she had sprung from. "Come along then miss I will walk you back to your room to make sure you get safely inside" she told him the room number then proceeded to direct him "I know where it is madam I work here" he told her wondering to himself had she been sleepwalking or up to no good?
Another incident that the night porter on duty got confronted with was the guest who had arrived earlier that day gone up to the rooms where the housekeepers were working and dumped his possessions in a bedroom not even bothering to check in first just selecting a room of his choice, he was attending a wedding downstairs on the premises, later that evening after drinking and smoking weed he approached the reception desk to ask for a key to his room, by now he had no idea that the room key he was given was a totally different room to the one he had plonked himself in earlier that day, he proceeded upstairs to the room number given him by the
 night porter only to find nothing his luggage was missing, he went back to reception where he started

accusing the night porter of stealing his weed (that's all he was bothered about) it got pretty heated so the police was called he was then arrested for possession of narcotics result!

The night staff also had to contend with the customers who had gone into the wrong room where other residents were installed insisting it was their room, arguments broke out causing the other rooms to pop their heads out to see what was going off, sometimes it was computer error (or staff not putting correct information in) or drunken, confused people who got disorientated with all the rooms and corridors looking alike. Nightmare for the evening staff to sort out.

This Hotel also had on site leisure facilities for guests and staff, Sauna, Steam room, Jacuzzi, pool, Gym and a Spa treatment room, somewhere to relax after a stressful day or a long tiring journey, or as a special treat for any occasion where you could include an afternoon tea in the bar lounge area. Very popular for Hen parties, Birthdays, Mother's Day anything you want to celebrate.

Now as you can imagine the staff in the pool area saw some sights, people are very vain, posing (look at me) which the guest wanted everyone to admire their physic, after all they had little clothes on, the elderly were probably the worst, one such gentleman would parade in the tiniest, skimpiest, tightest trunks you could imagine, he was very well endowed, (lucky man) of course your eyes were instantly diverted to this area which was the desired effect causing the young ones to go into fits of extreme laughter (not in front of the guest) then along came the elderly man which we call one ball Harry, yes its true, Tasha and Mark were keeping an eye on the pool area when they saw Harry walking towards them in his swim wear. "What's that hanging down in front of Harry" said Tasha trying not to giggle "I'm not sure" replied mark "It can't be can it" implied Tasha "I think it is" laughed Mark, Harrys swimwear had developed a hole where his testicle was located and it was the perfect fit for it to drop through(must have been gravity) obviously he was unaware (or was he) Mark and Tasha found it very hard to keep their composure as soon as they were out of sight they fell about laughing.

 I mean what can you say it's not something you can bring to his attention now is it? Another incident which is widely talked about is the time Nic the evening lifeguard caught a couple after having a late-night swim actually having sex in the pool, they obviously could not wait must have been something in the water. Things will always happen unexpectedly which are out of our control which catches us out on the hop. A busy afternoon in the gym and pool area was running smoothly until without warning all the power cut out.

 The young lady who was put in charge of the department and alone on shift realised that she needed to evacuate all the members as everything was plunged into darkness, the pool area was to be the most challenging as it involved making sure everyone got out of the pool safely, also the steam room and jacuzzi, getting people to the changing rooms was very daunting with only the help of a torch some of the elderly ones wanted to stay put hoping to wait it out they were very stubborn, trying to tell them it wasn't safe and slowly helping them making sure they did not slip was hard work.

The Whole hotel and the surrounding areas were in a major power outage with no time scale of when it would be up and running the emergency generators had to be put in use. Thankfully it didn't happen often. Another great tradition of the hotel was when a staff member was moving on to other employment especially if they had given a long service it was the dunking! At the end of their final day their close team-mates threw them fully clothed in the pool, hopefully they could swim.

STEPPING DOWN

After my disastrous time serving as a housekeeping supervisor for the past year apparently not full- filling my duties to the correct standards of which I was totally unaware of I embarked on my new position as a breakfast team member in the large restaurant, very daunting, lots to learn. I had never done waitressing to this extent the only plus side was that I knew a lot of the staff so at least they could show me the ropes. It was a big change for me as I now was just an ordinary employee awaiting my orders, each supervisor, shift leader did it different which was very confusing to say the least I was at the other end of the spectrum so was always getting shouted at, I used to be at the top, not anymore although it was my choosing I just could not deal with all the conflict, to just get the job done to the best of my ability and go home without any stress was all I wanted.

I presumed that my work was fine although it was hard balancing all the crockery and cutlery which the others made it look easy, to me they were very heavy and slippery the knifes were forever falling off the plates, plus my confidence had taken a bashing and confronting customers face to face trying to remember what they had requested got me so confused I often took them the wrong order which didn't go down too well. Some of the guests got very impatient (probably got out the wrong side of bed) I just couldn't seem to grasp it, on top of all this I had the kitchen to navigate, the irate chefs who acted like a certain well known celebrity famous for his foul mouthed obscenity's not very patient with new staff, you were an encumbrance! then there was   the pot washers, (kitchen porters) or KP's for short all telling you not to do this and that, plus it was hot and smelly, and I was always burning my fingers, everything seemed so heavy. I wondered if I had made the right choice asking to step down. I did not have a lot of options at the time as I was very ill so could not perform to the best of my ability in my previous role; I presumed this position would be less stressful with not being in charge. How wrong can a person be? My memory was slipping fast as the disease was taking hold, I was having great difficulty trying to keep up, one day everything was fine then on my next shift my mind would be totally blank. I eventually went off sick for 17 months as I was recovering from major brain surgery to remove a tumour which if had not been found was shortening my life. Everything now made sense as to why my work performance was going downhill, my memory was being destroyed.

On my return to work I simply had to relearn everything again from scratch, I progressed quite quickly with the help of my team mates some of the staff had been replaced which made it easier for me as we were all on the same level which made it not so daunting. It was very hard and frightening starting again, I was nervous, afraid, it is a customer facing job and I didn't want to make a fool of myself, and because I was more mature people expect you to have a certain level of experience so would turn to me for answers, I did make a lot of mistakes especially with the taking of payments, I just couldn't seem to grasp it, just got to keep on practising.

The guests still had their dirty habits, very demanding and greedy, they would pile up their plates knowing full well that they wouldn't be able to eat it all but as it was a buffet they wanted their money's worth, ordering extra's from the a la carte menu on the table mostly the free items, but the mess they left behind was disgusting, I'm sure that it would not happen in their own homes, as they were paying and didn't have to clean up so be it! It was the baked beans, scrambled egg and the pastries that got everywhere always squashed in the carpet plus people would put dollops of tomato sauce on their plates which would get all over your fingers when removing them.

 I would be embarrassed walking away from the table letting everyone think I was a pig! The families did not set very good examples especially with the babies in the high chairs they would let their little darlings squash food all over and onto the floor never dreaming to pick it up, no; they would just walk away and leave the mess for the next person to sit in.

Not all the people were nice some were very rude and did not have any manners looking down on us, but we waiters and waitresses get our revenge behind the scenes never underestimate us, we are the people who serve you, we are human and like many places what goes on behind closed doors stays behind closed doors. We will smile graciously and accommodate your every demand until we get into the kitchen where we will vent our anger at you, say a few choice words, let our colleagues know what you are really like then return to your table with the utmost professionalism.

My team mates consisted of all ages, both sexes, we all bonded together each bringing something different to the table, we would laugh, joke, poke fun at each other sometimes we would bicker, get bitchy, especially when we were rushed off our feet, we got tired, mardy, it was a very tiring job, running up and down, in and out of the kitchen carrying heavy trays of dirty plates, glasses, mugs and cutlery we just did not have time to stop even to go to the loo until it was near the end of service.

Our tempers were frayed, we were sweaty, thirsty, some staff did not pull their weight they walked as if they had all the time in the world, most frustrating to say the least, it was different generations that were paid peanuts so had no intention of breaking into a sweat couldn't blame them it wasn't really their cup of tea they were used to doing evenings working in banqueting, they would lay the tables back to front even after being employed in the industry for the past 6 months, the supervisor would shout at them, I laughed, I loved the younger ones they were more exciting, nothing bothered them except playing on their smart phones and partying it reminded me of my younger days, carefree, looking forward to the future after all they were not going to do this type of work forever it was just a stop gap earning them some spends while studying.

We had a check list to mark off the guests as they entered the restaurant, the more experienced staff would do all the patter but some of the younger ones were a little curt leaving the guest to fend for themselves which didn't go down very good especially with the well to do ones, we would show them over and over it was experience and confidence which was lacking.

Now me I had memory problems with remembering the young ones names even though they had badges on they all looked the same to me they found this highly amusing so they answered to whatever I called them, I was always teasing them and singing to them I'm sure they thought I was going senile maybe I am?

One thing that makes my job worthwhile is they always ask me if they are not sure of anything as I am easy to approach and don't snap at them, in fact I show them rather than tell them so they can have a go themselves.

We all have to start somewhere but some of the staff would get peed off with them as would the guests.

The business men liked being served by the young ladies after all it was a bit of eye candy first thing in the morning, but the more mature visitors liked pampering and reminiscing so were harder work especially if they thought a freebie was coming their way, and boy did they try.

Then came the residents with food allergies, Gluten free, Vegan, Vegetarian, Nut, Dairy, things we didn't know off, that's fine I hear you say so why do these people not know what they can and cannot eat?

Yes unbelievable, we do cater for all and we can adapt, one incident happened on an exceptionally busy shift I was working alone on the hot buffet trying to keep it full when a lady confronted me over the hot pass and informed me that she was a vegetarian could she order some veggie sausages," yes of course" I replied "they take 10 mins to cook" that was fine, she then shouted in my face "what can I eat then" "Oh and I cannot have eggs" "well omelette is out of the question then" I muttered, I was hot, sweaty, knackered and had been running in and out for the last 4 hours non-stop, I reeled off the tomatoes, mushrooms, baked beans," have you any hash browns" she said "unfortunately we have run out of those" I told her so that wasn't an option, neither was the black pudding, "so what else can I have then?" she screamed at me (bearing in mind we had fruit, toast, cereals, pastries and such) I don't know what came over me I blurted out" bacon" "Is that not meat"? she was very angry now "yes" I replied "its pork" I made a hasty retreat into the kitchen huffing and cuffing she had drove me mad.

I then realised what I had said we all fell about laughing, surely you damn well know what you can consume if you are eating away from home?

Our lovely supervisor Samantha was not exempt from the customers outrages, one busy weekend shift a middle aged couple came into the restaurant for breakfast, it was not included in their room rate, Sam informed them of the pricing when the gentleman disagreed with the price saying "No its £10 not £12.50" his wife said "Just leave it, its ok" they paid and Sam took them to their table, everything was fine until his daughter and partner turned up for their breakfast and sat with them. Sam went over to explain things and the pricing, the gentleman spoke out "Its fine its paid for" "no sir" said Sam " only yours" well he jumped up like a man possessed shouting "what's going on here" clenching his fists looking as though he was going to punch Sam, sticking out his chest and invading Sam's space very threatening, Sam got very scared and squealed running off to reception very upset, she told the Duty Manager what had happened and that she didn't feel safe, she came back into the restaurant got their money out of the till and told them to leave she wasn't happy with his behaviour and she didn't want him in the restaurant anymore, she was in her rights to do so as no one should feel threatened when doing their job.

His family were very upset with him as he had spoilt their breakfast and ironically, it turned out that he was a teacher at that.

Summer time always threw up problems in the restaurant one was the excessive heat even though it had air- con it didn't seem to work, we had large floor to ceiling windows that would draw the sun, it was like working in a green-house boy did we sweat, in fact we melted, running up and down didn't help.

It also attracted lots of flies no matter what we used we could just not get rid of them, the exterminators provided all-sorts but the little devils out foxed them, swatting them with the oven cloths (when the guests were not looking) was our favourite past-time, you have to laugh we pretended that we couldn't see them when the customers were there it was as though we were oblivious to them yet we could see them landing on the food (dirty bloody things) we did try to cover as much as possible.

The best part was when the restaurant closed; we would spray the fly repellent talk about killing the damn things we would choke on the bloody fumes. One of the waitresses was forever opening the fire door to let in some air, she was always in trouble as the manager said it stopped the air-con working, but we didn't think it worked in the first place. The staff canteen was also a no go area that too was under fire from the flies, all the windows and doors had to remain closed which made it like an oven, they even had fly papers hanging down above your head while you was trying to get some food not really a nice experience. Can you imagine how many slipped off and into the food? Protein? I for one am glad we don't get time for breaks working in the restaurant.

The maintenance team was quite large in this hotel after all there was always lots to do be it plumbing, electrics, repairs especially after large events, decorating, room maintenance such as guests getting locked in the bathrooms, in fact any issue that was thrown at them from all departments it was a very demanding job, the team consisted of young and more mature guys one in particular was a torment a ladies man (so he thinks) never wrong, always got an answer, a proper bob the builder type guy always wanting freebies like a bacon butty and coffee, sometimes a pain in the bum, he would make you laugh and get frustrated but at least he was a friendly sort. If you happened to be hoovering the restaurant, he would switch off your appliance when passing making you think that the hoover had cut out, he must have had a fetish with plug sockets.

 The younger ones liked to converse with the young ladies, exchanging banter and such after all we all worked in the same building so team spirit was a must. The Granddaddy of the team was the one that put us all in our places often telling us off about not doing the correct things which we all need at times just to keep us level-headed, and of course for our well-being and safety.

One day that will always hold special memories in our hearts was the sad news of the death of one of our dearly loved colleagues' who will always be missed.
Her name was Elaine she was a character in her own rights, she had worked for the company for 11 years, her role was that of early morning cleaner with her best friend who looked after all the public areas amongst many other duties always willing to lend a hand to

whoever needed her, it was such a shock that someone so young would be taken away from us so suddenly we just could not believe it, and it was the start of her holiday which she had longingly been looking forward to so unfair. We all have our own memories of her, but she will be remembered for her liking of her famous earmuffs which were placed on her coffin, she probably wore them to block us out.

FUNCTIONS

We are a large hotel with a few function rooms that can accommodate your Special occasions, Weddings, Funerals, Baby showers, Birthday parties, Conference Lunch, School Prom in fact anything you want to celebrate. The biggest events were the Indian Weddings WOW! They were spectacular no expense spared, very opulent, like a scene from Bollywood, Beautiful dresses, Transport, such as Limousines, sports cars, horse and carriage you name it they got it, and guests in their hundred's where did all these people come from? Coach loads, I would not have known so many people in my lifetime if I tried.

They had Drummers, Dancers, Photographers, Fireworks (even though they were not allowed) we were located near a duel carriage way so the smoke effect would blind the drivers, not to be deterred they lit them anyway.

Gowns bedecked with jewels to die for and their own caterers who fessed up round the back of the hotel with their big vats of curries sat there heating them up, the aroma was delicious if you liked that sort of food, they would take over half of the big hotel kitchen cooking all sorts of delicious spicy food.

I would always ask for a morsel if on shift and they were very lovely people who loved for you to try some, it tasted nothing like the Indian takeaways. They didn't drink Alcohol so had gallons of fizzy bottles of coke, orange etc. The celebratory arrival drink was placed on tables in front of the entrance these consisted of fruit juices and the massive chocolate fountains, YUM, YUM. The downside was the mess after the wedding was over you have never seen anything like it, after all a room with over 1000 people all eating and drinking was a massive challenge, we were quite adapt at clearing up although it took many of us quite a substantial time to put it back to some semblance.

The public toilets were the worst with lots of paper towels, toilet rolls, nappies, glasses, bottles, paper plates, confetti and blocked toilets unable to cope with the huge demand, not a job for the faint hearted.

The English weddings were the most destructive, large gatherings of drink fuelled adults often resulting in fighting would smash the fittings off the walls, the toilet doors took a battering as well as some guests, the tables and chairs would get involved lovely times?

I would assume they had paid a bond after all the management knew what to expect.

Conferences were a regular feature with people congregating from around the world they would have lots of tea breaks, buffet lunch which could carry on for a few days, famous celebrities would sometimes appear often with merchandise for sale it was the porters that got the running around jobs, nonstop work very exhausting constantly refilling tea and coffee.

Christmas Day was another massive event booked up way before the big day, the dinner was served in all 3 rooms, the big ballroom was a huge hot buffet, the smaller function room was a more compact version but the biggest was table service in the restaurant, lots of entertainment provided, Magician, Balloon maker, pianist, and of course the big man himself Santa, he had his own Grotto in the reception area. It was a military operation staff were not allowed to book this time of year off as we needed as many hands to the decks as possible, any one that works in hospitality hates this time of year, yes it's a good atmosphere out front but behind the scenes we are all knackered, stressed, shouting at each other.

The meals are all plated up and stored in racks in the ovens so when it's time to serve them they are bloody hot, no amount of gloves stops the plates from burning you we run in with them like carrying hot coals ready to throw them at you especially when your manager is trying to direct you to the correct table and they are going too slow, you want to shout hurry up my fingers are on fire, its natural instinct to let go when you've reached your threshold, it's the worst part of the job.

I wonder how many staff have done just that. Then you get the guest who has forgotten what they ordered many months ago and leave you balancing the burning plate until they decide what it was, or worse still refuse to accept it and you have to return it to the kitchen. The best part of the day is after we have turned the restaurant around from breakfast to the festive lunch we have a little breather to celebrate with a glass of prosecco and our famous secret Santa unwrapping, that's our Christmas until we get home and crash ready for the next day, too exhausted to do anything else. After serving all those Christmas Dinners it's the last thing you want, I usually have a bacon sandwich, chocolate and a Guinness for energy.

Another large event was the Annual staff party, this also included staff from our sister hotels so was quite a large turnout, it was usually held after the festive season when we had a quieter period, we got to see some of our old friends who had moved around.

It had a theme, entertainment, free booze and food, awards and the disco. It was to say thank you for all our hard work, the younger ones would go off to the city to party all night long.

The managers also had their nights of letting their hair down most of them choose to stay overnight so as not to drink and drive, that was like a green light to get rat-arsed and they sure did.

One talked about incident happened after a heavy session the poor night manager had the problem to deal with, One of the big boys decided that he would take a stroll along the corridor completely starkers, he was obviously unaware of where he was probably believing that he was at home and needed the bathroom, it's a good job none of the guests were around then it would have been a disaster. The night manager had to coax him back into his room which was quite a challenge, after the news circulated around the staff we all had our own ideas of what he was up to, we laughed and told jokes, even singing songs related to having no clothes on, it kept us amused for a little while until another event happened.

PRESENT DAY

Well after many years of business the management are embarking on a new venture will it be successful one can only hope, the restaurant is having a makeover and being transformed into a well-known famous top chef steak house and grill, lots of new staff all trained before they are allowed to work in there, new fixtures and fittings, new opening times, new kitchen appliances and lots of teething problems. Here say is rife about what's going on who is working where and when, are staff going to be moved to other hotels in the group, lots of gossip which always happens in these situations and a new General Manager to come on board.

Then you have the guests, some will hate it some will love it after all you cannot please everyone.

Some people do not like change including staff; it's the unknown that puts them off. We had by now moved the temporary restaurant into the nearest available function room, it was a Saturday in June when weddings were rife, so space was an issue.

This day, two events were taking place, the smaller room had a removable wall partition so we could split it into two, the smaller side was set up for the marriage ceremony while the other half was prepared for the wedding breakfast, all was going well until a couple of the staff were putting stock in place for the next morning's breakfast when the young lady knocked over the kitchen cloths barrow narrowly missing dropping the glass flower vases on the floor, unbeknown to them the couple were saying their vows at the place where the registrar says "If anyone knows of any reason why these two should not be joined in matrimony speak now" when Josephine shouts to the young lady "What yer doing" she couldn't have timed it better. The supervisor Sandra came running out playing hell saying" be quiet will you there's a wedding taking place everyone can hear you" we all fell about laughing in the kitchen what's the chance of that happening at the crucial moment?

Maybe it's an omen? The guests were not impressed with the temporary place for breakfast we started getting lots of complaints that it's not good enough, the plates are not warm, we have a plate warmer in the actual restaurant but obviously it's out of bounds so we just have to make do but no people love to moan we are doing the best we can, we the staff are finding it stressful it's like having a pop up shop always on the move, we ourselves don't know where the supplies have been moved too, we are working extra hours to sort things out.

Lucy came into the kitchen ranting saying "would they like to get up at 4am to warm the f---ing plates you don't do it at home, that woman's just screamed in my face, stupid cow". It's hard keeping your feelings to yourself they have no idea how much effort we put in.

The majority of staff, some newbies as well were on their training for the new restaurant lots to remember but interesting to see what the new lay-out was going to look like, it was getting exciting as time was drawing nearer to the grand opening, nerves were kicking in, the kitchen also were undergoing a vast training programme lots of activity all around.

Staff and guests were getting stressed with one another, we were under a lot of pressure in a small confined space it would have been easier if the customers were staggered when coming down for breakfast in an ideal world, but no they all came together which caused immense problems, not enough seating, not enough food, no matter how hard we tried we just could not keep up, tempers frayed, accidents occurring, what a nightmare! The day finally arrived when we got to go back to our home boy had we missed it, the restaurant looked very impressive with its new colour scheme and grand fittings, the smell of new carpet which lingers for a while made it all the more fresher but was a bugger to hoover, in fact the amount of bum fluff that came away I could have made myself a new carpet for home. Everything was getting sorted until it came to the change over from breakfast to Steakhouse that's when it was apparent that this was not going to be as straight forward as we anticipated, we the breakfast staff had to do the initial table set up but like all Hotels staff shortage was a big issue lots more were needed.

It was the same old same old and we were exhausted after doing breakfast then to have a timescale put on you is no easy feat, we just could not keep up it was so tiring, our other duties were falling beside the way side guests were complaining as all the focus was on the new venture, hopefully with time and repetitiveness it will get better.

When the trainers have departed, it's like having big brother watching your every move, things will settle down, some of the staff will not make it and quit it happens. After the first full week, long hours, lots of new routines to adapt to we were all getting a little flustered tiredness was kicking in our tempers were short it wouldn't take long to light the fuse then bang!

This happened on the next busy Saturday we were extremely busy, the customers kept coming and coming no let up, it was the hottest day of the year so far when Lucy who filled up the hot buffet breakfast food had an altercation with the Head Chef both fiery ladies, they were going at it hell for leather screaming at each other all over the quantity of the fried eggs, Lucy shouting in Mary's face " Why can't you cook more than 4\6 eggs at once, it's not enough" "Don't you shout at me telling me what I can and cannot do, I'm doing my best I am on my own in here, I've got eggs in the pan look" replied Mary "Well I've had enough of you shouting at me I'm scared of asking for stuff it's like walking on egg shells" said Lucy marching off leaving a fuming Mary chuntering away, the next minute Lucy marched back in proclaiming that she was out of here gathering all her belongings screaming obscenities.

We all just stopped and stared wondering what on earth had just happened?

Sandra our supervisor shouted" Carry on we have lots of guests out front" we just marched around like tin pot soldiers stunned wondering if Lucy had quit? After a short while she returned and carried on as if nothing had happened it was surreal. It was not just staff losing it we were used to having the police called to the hotel of a night time but this was breakfast time on a lovely sunny day when the Gardeners were busy at work their van parked out front with the doors open when along comes a police riot van and an ambulance, the big bushes did obscure the view somewhat the guests were asking "What's going on?" we were just as clueless "No idea" I replied to one nosy customer "Maybe the gardener chopped his arm off" he dramatized people like a drama! "Why don't you go out and look" I said "Oh no that would be too nosy" he answered back then my colleague called me in the kitchen "You will never guess what's happened out front" she seemed quite amused " This chap who is a bit of a loud mouth had an altercation with a fellow resident over car-parking it resulted in the Guest decking the loud mouth, as he fell backwards banging his head on concrete he lost consciousness so an ambulance was called which resulted in the police attending" Now that's what I call road rage! Entertainment for the customers while having breakfast, you cannot make it all up.

We must not forget our regular guests some of which stay on a long-term basis, we are on first name terms with the majority and likewise it's like having family stay. They have their own special requirements and love our friendly banter with each other it makes our job worthwhile, when their companies move them on its like losing a friend, we have met some lovely people which we try our best to make them feel at home especially as they are away from their loved ones, a friendly face makes all the difference.

Now we all know that the customer is always right or so they think, now things are settling back down the residents are now back to their normal selves of complaining no matter how much we do for them, along comes what we presume are a lovely elderly couple with mobility problems, I greet them, take them over to a suitable table near the buffet breakfast ask all the relevant questions and make sure that all their needs are catered for going the extra mile, nothing is too much trouble, I ask the lady who is in a motorized chair if she is staying in it or can she transfer to a dining chair with ease? "I will leave my scooter here if that's alright?" she answered which was a couple of feet away down the corridor leading towards the kitchen.

She got out folded the chair up and walked over to the dining chair which I had pulled out for her no problems, I took their orders and went about my duties, on returning Josephine the shift leader picked it up and removed it to the other side so no one would fall over it, well the elderly gentleman jumped out of his chair and proceeded to shout at Josephine that she should not have moved it and how on earth had she managed to fold it up, he was very abrupt in his manner insinuating that Josephine had probably broke it and he needed to start it up to check it, I intervened and told him his good lady wife had collapsed it herself when she exited it, he then proceeded to take the scooter back to their table as he obviously did not trust us, that's what we get for being nice to folk how wrong can one be?

It must have been a day of complainers as the next customers who arrived just as we were closing were the guests from who knows where talk about demanding, just because they had more points they assumed that they were above anyone else and we were their personal slaves, they ordered everything even though breakfast had finished making us run in and out of the kitchen umpteen times, their table was laden with enough food for the entire day, then disaster struck, a little black fly appeared and spoilt it all well that was it they couldn't possibly eat anything now, we did apologize it is summer after all, then to top it all off they happened to see a large rodent scoot across the carpark, well they would, we are situated in a large green wooded area ideal for pests looking for their next meal, that was the final straw they upped and left probably never to return.

On another occasion three burly guys were sat having breakfast all looking out of the window towards the bushes as they had obviously spotted something that they did not expect to see, you guessed it, no it wasn't a rabbit or a squirrel it was our local friendly vermin, I could hear them tittering which was causing other guests to look so I went over asked if everything was alright, they proceeded to tell me what they had seen so trying to make light on the situation I bent down and whispered to them," you should only worry if you see ratatouille on the menu as you will know where it's come from" they all laughed and got on with their breakfast.

The most important thing in a Hotel is the last meal that a customer will remember, they will overlook a bit of dust, a missing towel, the cockup at check in, so it is very important that we provide a great breakfast, friendly staff members, making the guests wanting to return on a future visit, if they leave disgruntled we will more than likely get bad feedback and that's something none of us want. Things are now moving on staff leaving for new employment in other hotels, new employees joining the team, a wider variety of guests all eager to try the new restaurant including celebrities, promotions, filming, keeping us all very busy, even a new General Manager which fortunately we already know so hopefully he will get lots of support. I have just completed 10 years' service and to my greatest surprise I received a lovely monetary gift to say thank you which makes you feel very valued. This is Hotel life you either love it or hate it! We will never get it perfect all we can do is try!

ACKNOWLEDGEMENTS

I would like to firstly thank the Hospitality Action Charity who kindly supported me when I was recovering from my Brain Tumour operation, they took away the stresses making my return to work much smoother. The proceeds from the sales of this book are being donated to their -selves to help others in similar circumstances.
My work colleagues old and new who have supplied me with true events that they have witnessed or have been involved in personally, all names are fictious and in no way relate to them.
Also, my daughter for editing and designing the book cover which I am so grateful for, taking time out of her own busy schedule and supporting me.
Friends, Family, who have been my Guinea pigs helping me with research and keeping me grounded.

Printed in Great Britain
by Amazon